OSCAR OCEAN AND ' FEAST

JOSEPHINE N. C. GROENHART

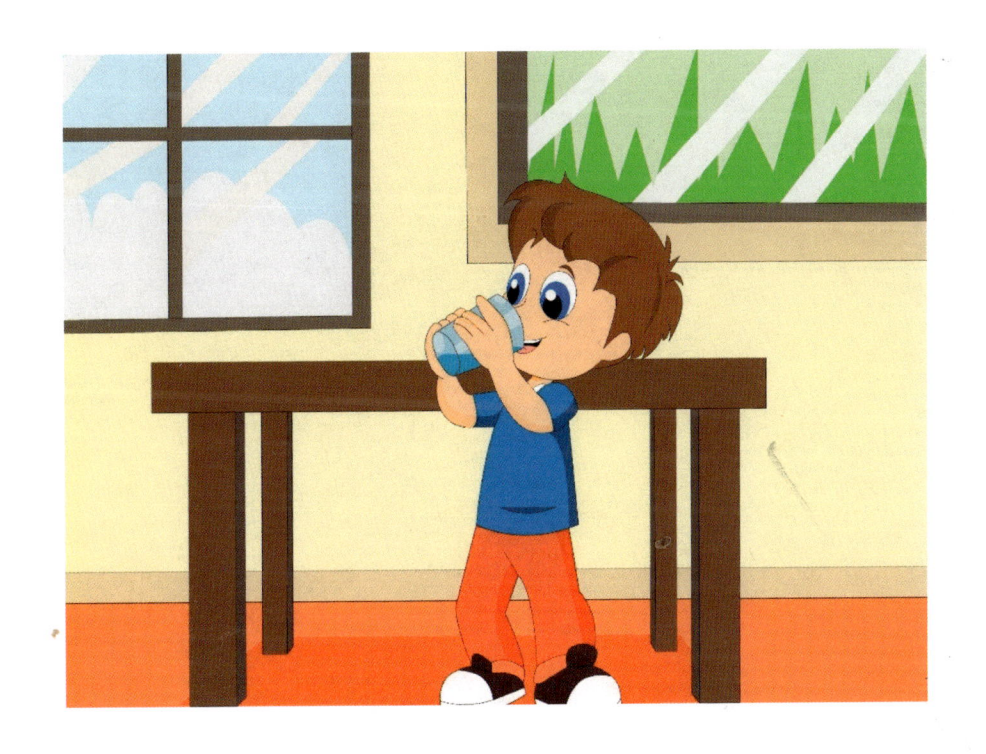

Copyright © 2016 Josephine N. C. Groenhart

All rights reserved.

ISBN:1508631646
ISBN-13: 978-1508631644

DEDICATION

For Isaac and Oakley. My two cheeky monkeys!

ACKNOWLEDGMENTS

With special thanks to Ambadi Kumar for her amazing illustrations, Ed for all your encouragement and Isaac, Oakley and all the children in our centre who have helped me put this together for you all.

THANK YOU

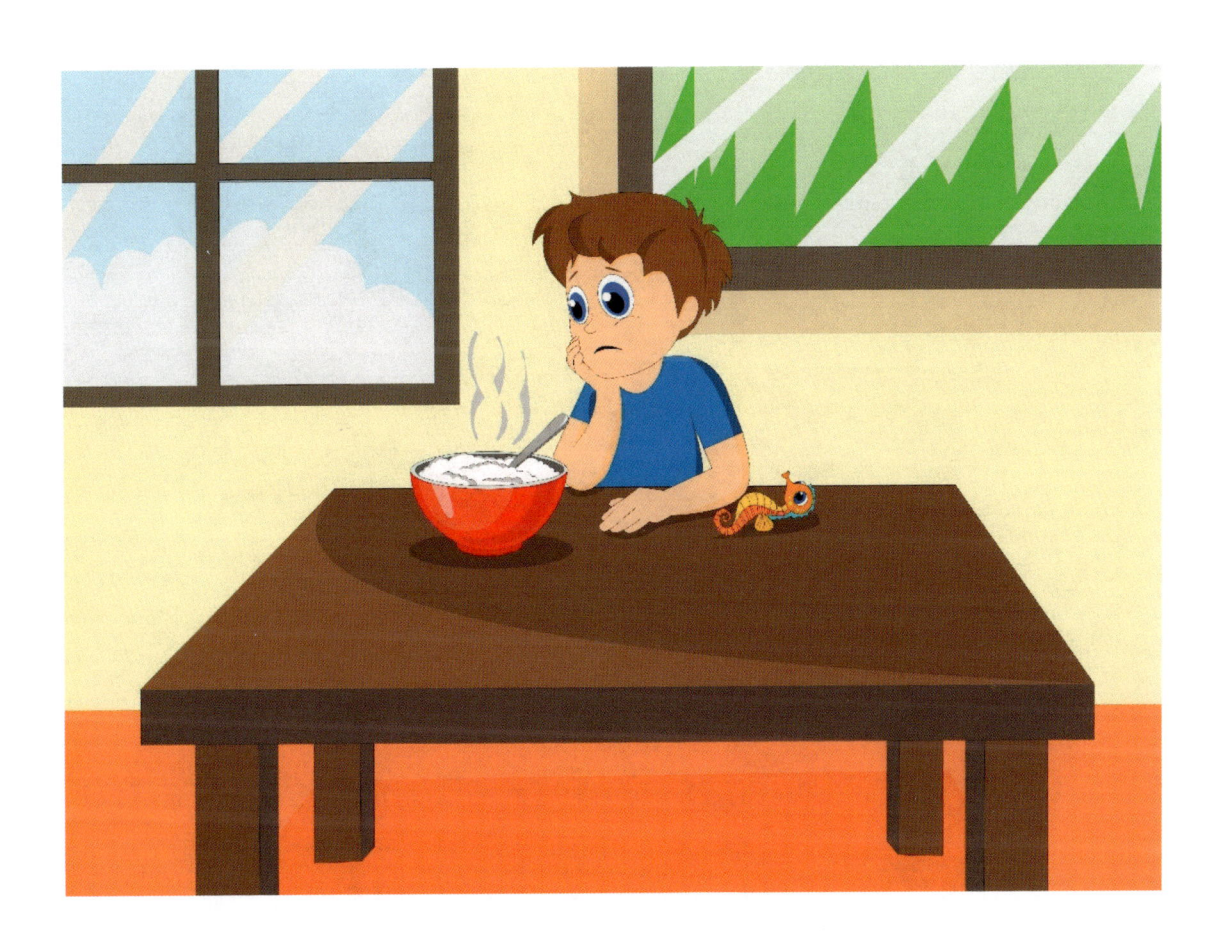

At breakfast Oscar simply shook his head

For mum had made muesli and Smoothie instead

"Eat up now Oscar and start this way,

For breakfast is the most important meal of the day."

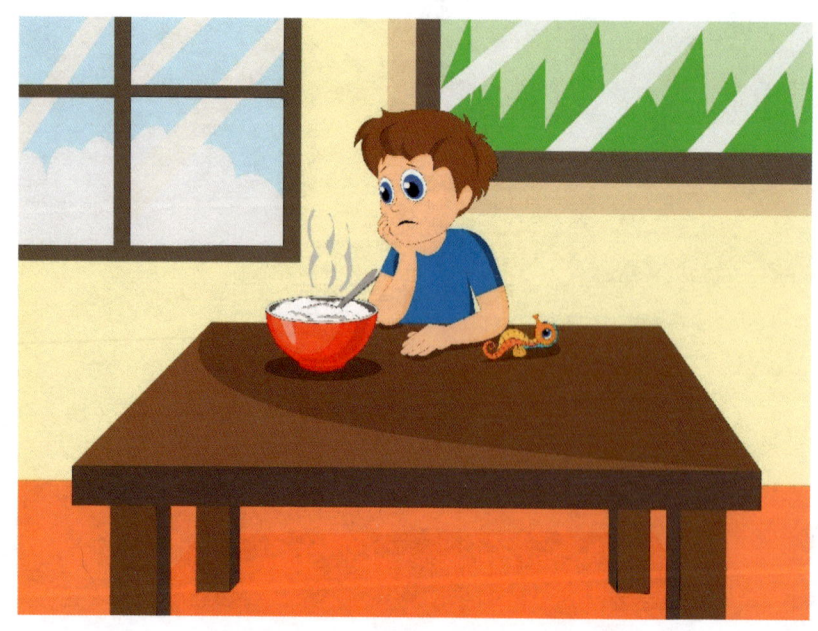

"I don't like that" Oscar said, pushing his plate firmly away

"Can't I have chocolate cereals, squash and then play?"

But mum was not listening; she was out in the hall

Busying and bustling, getting ready for pre-school

Wise young Sammy, in his big Chef hat:

"Come on Now Oscar, none of that,

If you want to grow big and wise and strong,

Nutrition is important all day long."

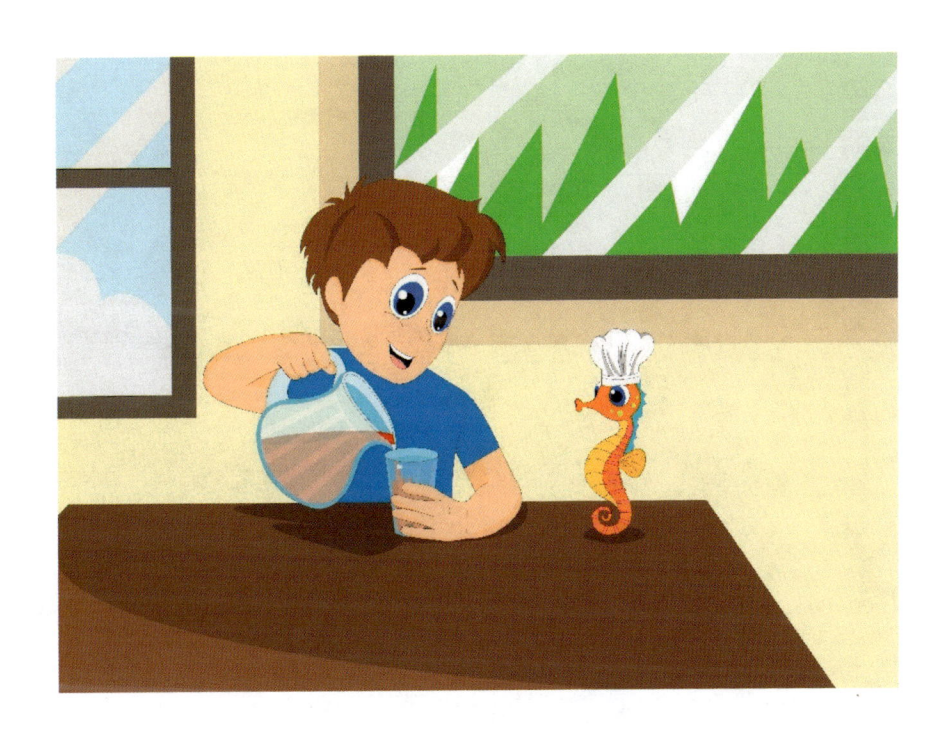

To Oscar it all sounded dull and boring

But a glass of Smoothie, Sammy was pouring.

"Packed full of vitamins, protein and water

Giving you energy, so you can be smarter."

"Let me introduce you Oscar to good basic Nutrition,"

Follow me closely, look hard and listen.

Your body needs food to heal, grow, and survive

The choice is yours if you want to thrive"

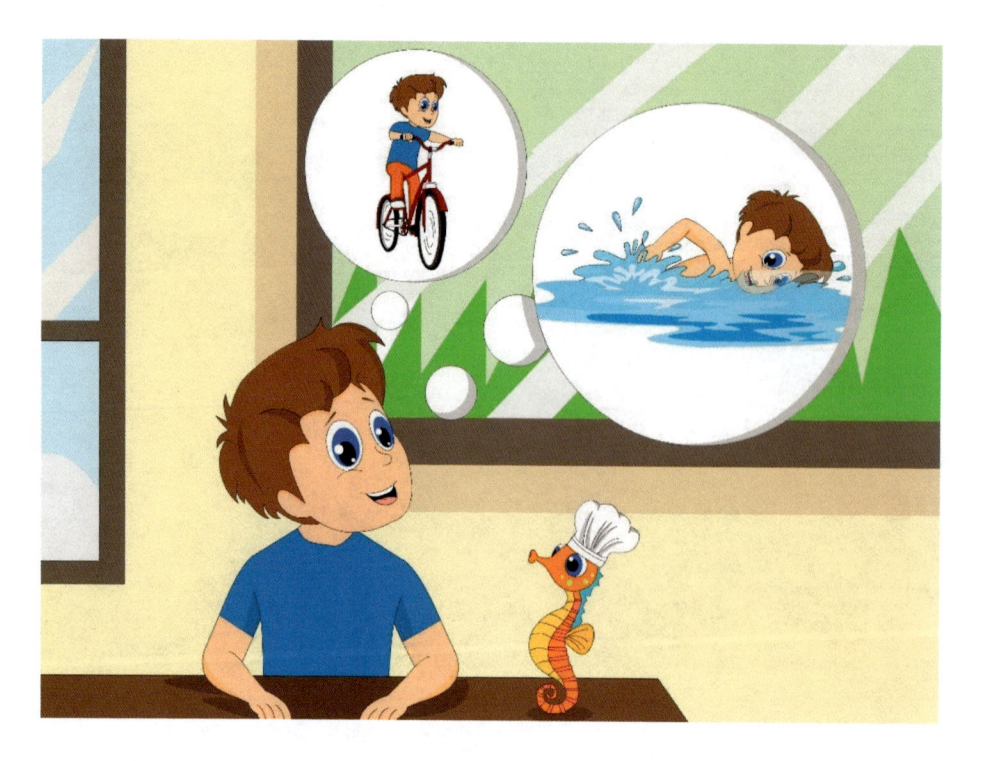

"Do you want to do lots of exciting things, like running and jumping;

Laughing, playing with friends, reading and swimming?

So come with me now and investigate food,

Some helpers we need; now where is the brood?"

Sidney Starfish appeared on Oscar's shoulder,

"Rule number one is drinking plenty of water."

Known as H-2-O it's great for hydration,

And very important for our brains to function."

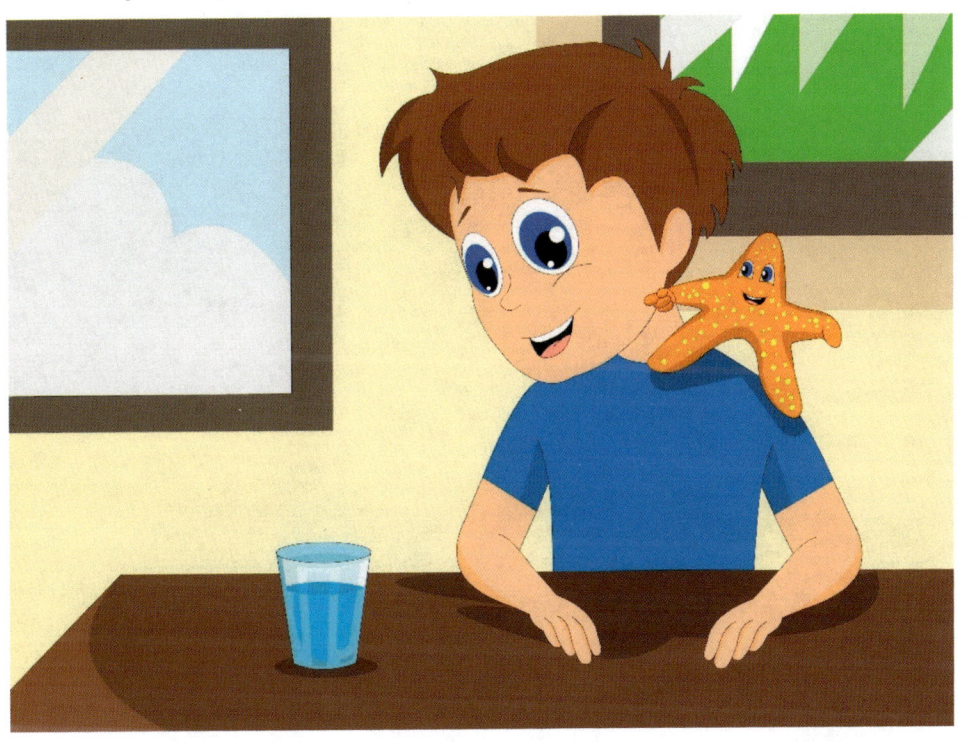

"Lack of water can cause your head to ache,

Your breath to smell and your knees to quake.

So drink plenty of water, Oscar, don't you stop

And very soon in the class you'll be top."

Drinking his water Oscar admitted it felt good,

He knew he must drink more, yes he should.

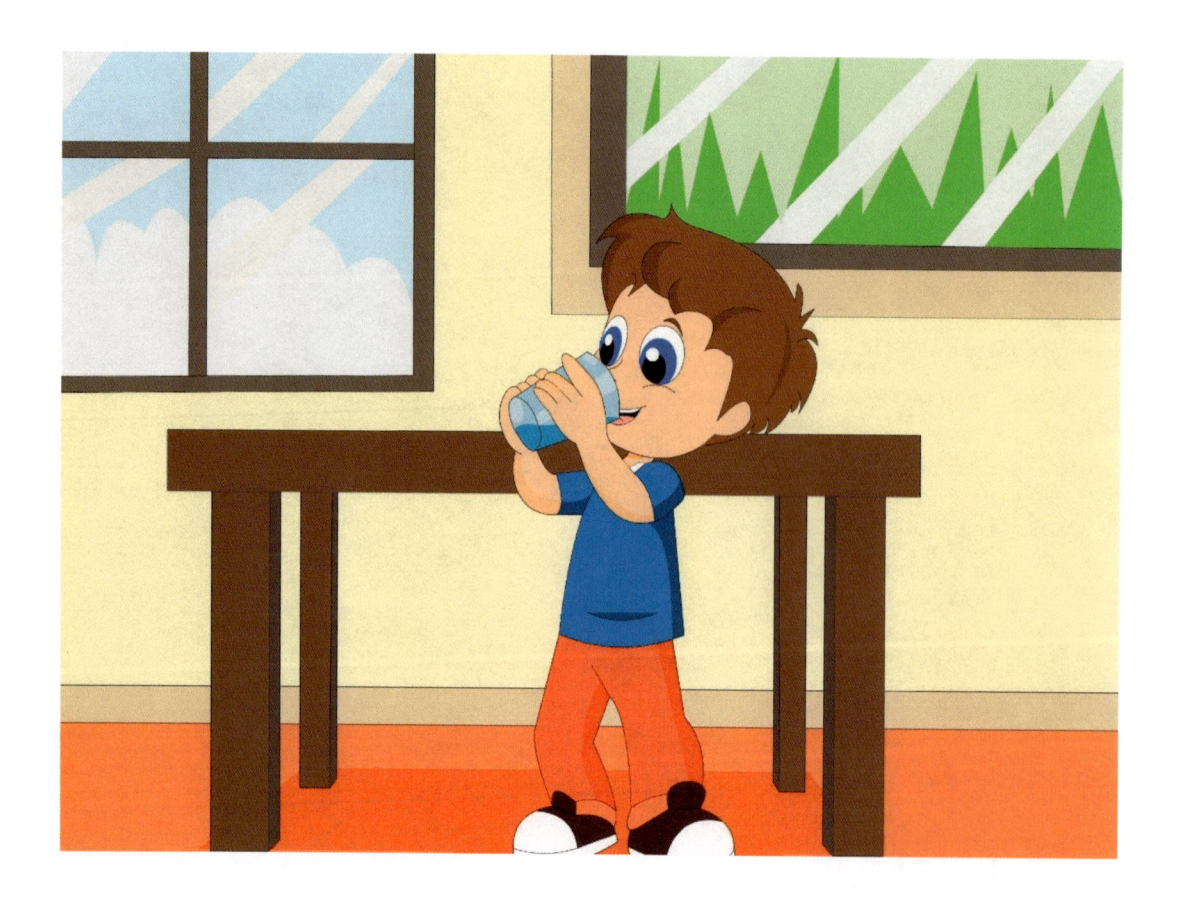

"Rule number two," Emily Eel did say

Peeling a banana as she slid his way

"Eat plenty of fruit, Oscar, different ones, too,

Apples, pears and oranges are all great for you.

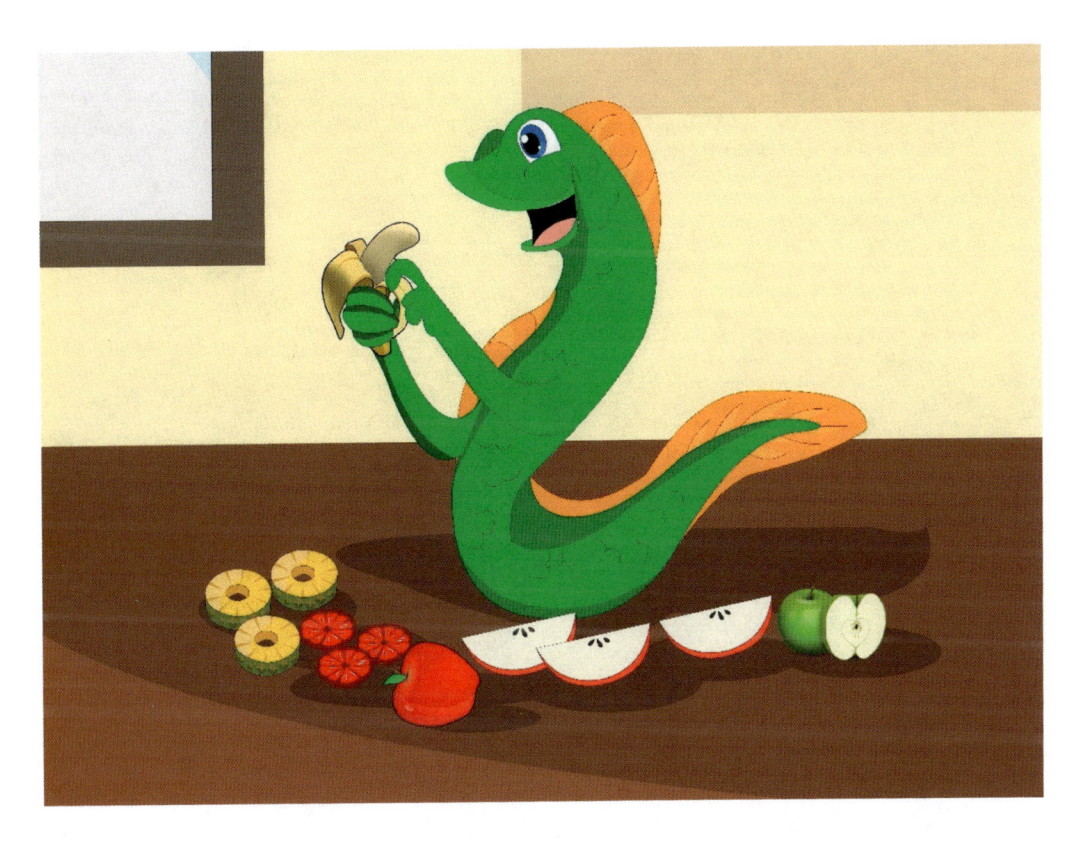

"There are so many different ones you can choose

With plenty of fruit you cannot lose,

The natural vitamins that they provide

Will help you feel amazing on the inside."

Opening the cupboard, and pulling out a parsnip

"With Rule Number Three, let us now equip."

Sammy Seahorse explained "load up with vegetables,

For you'll find they provide a multitude of minerals."

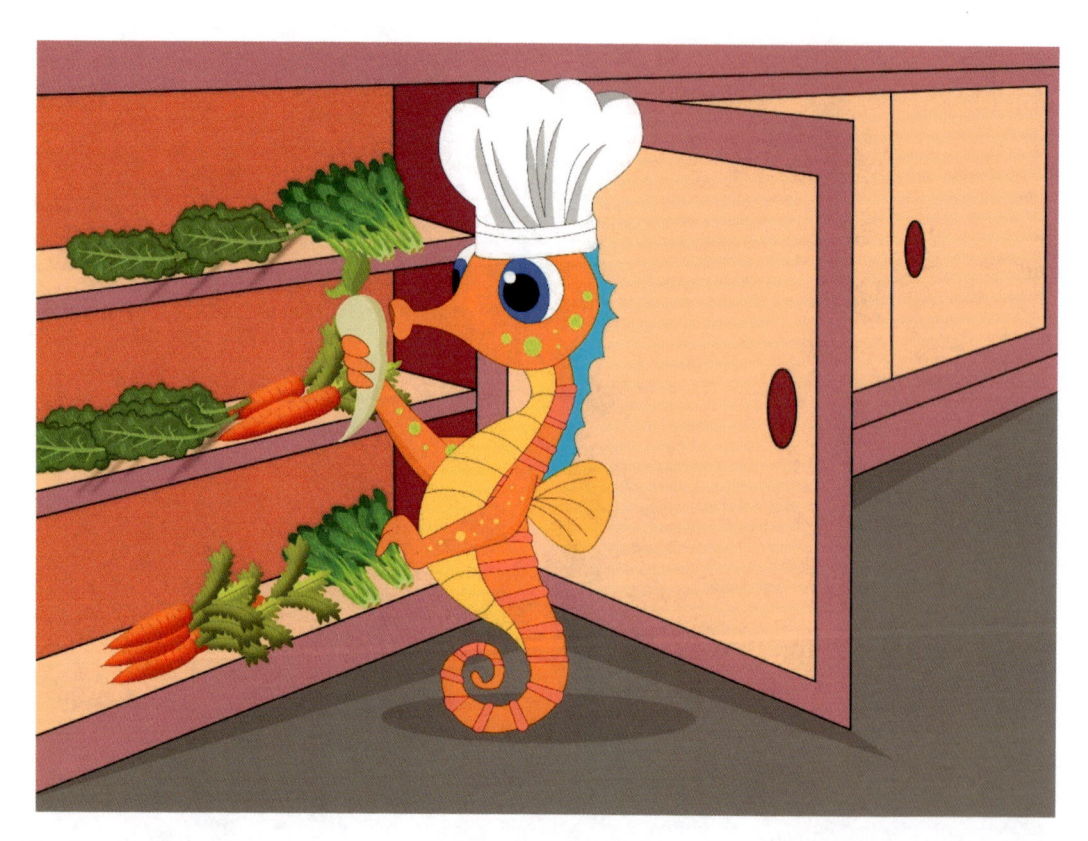

"There are so many fun veggies for you to eat,

Kale, spinach and carrots: oh Oscar, what a treat!

The iron they provide, to name one of so many,

Helps you to stay strong, not tired and like jelly."

Oscar smiled away for he began to see

How important fruit and veg was to stay healthy

"What would be next?", he wondered, wide-eyed

For Rule Number Four, Olga Urchin stood by his side:

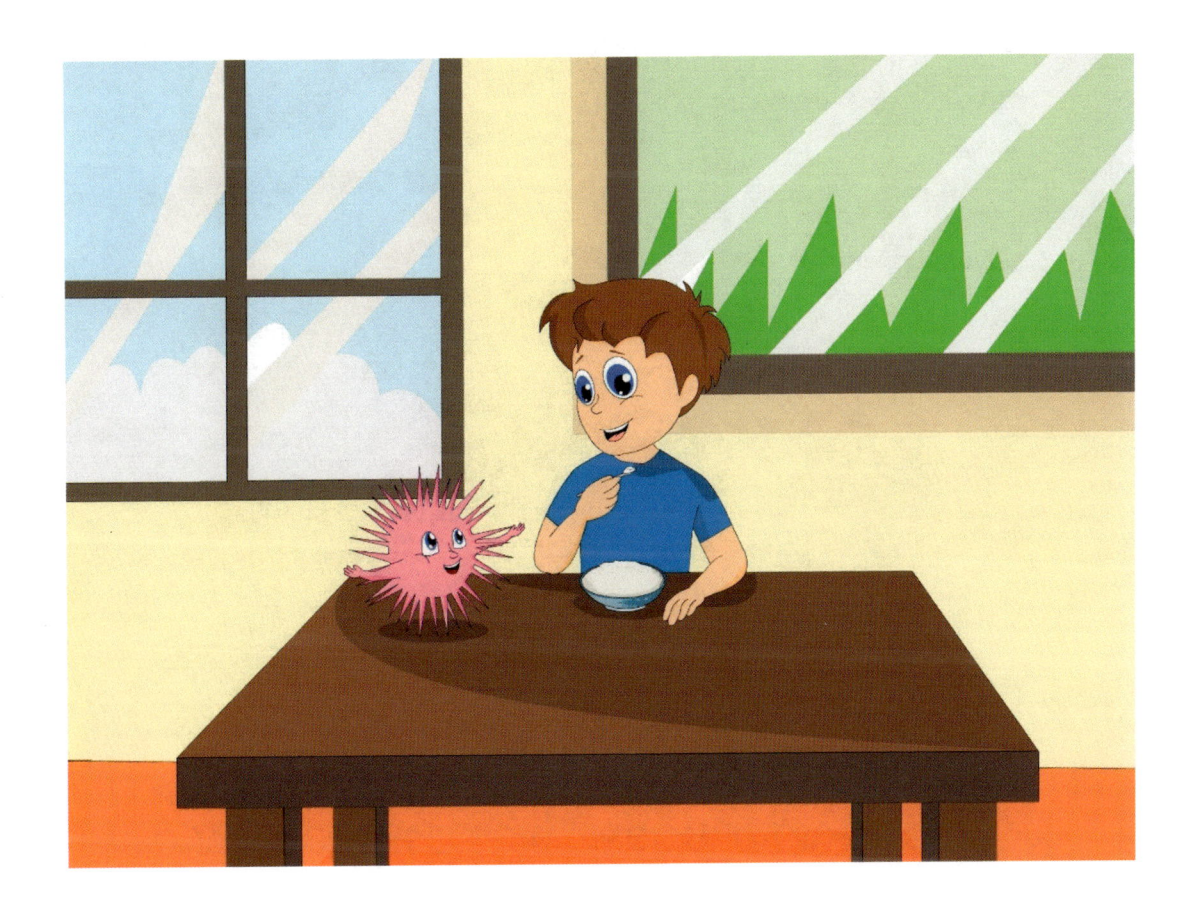

"Don't eat lots of junk", as told sternly by Olga:

"Avoid all those chips and that fast food burger.

There are so many naughties they pack in and hide

They may look good, but what's really inside?"

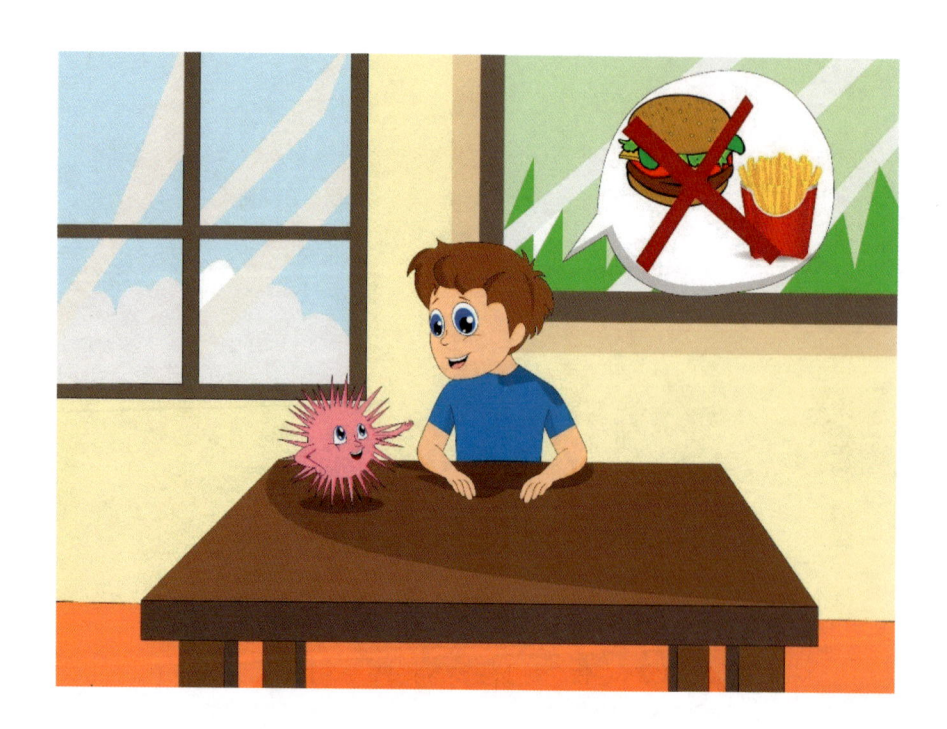

"Chemical preservatives - in they all go -

Doing what to your body? No one really knows."

Eating too much junk and processed fatty food

Can make us all ill and in a foul mood."

"So choose you food wisely." Olga did say.

"I always aim to think of it this way,

My body is a temple, but if it were a car,

And I put in the wrong fuel, it would not get far."

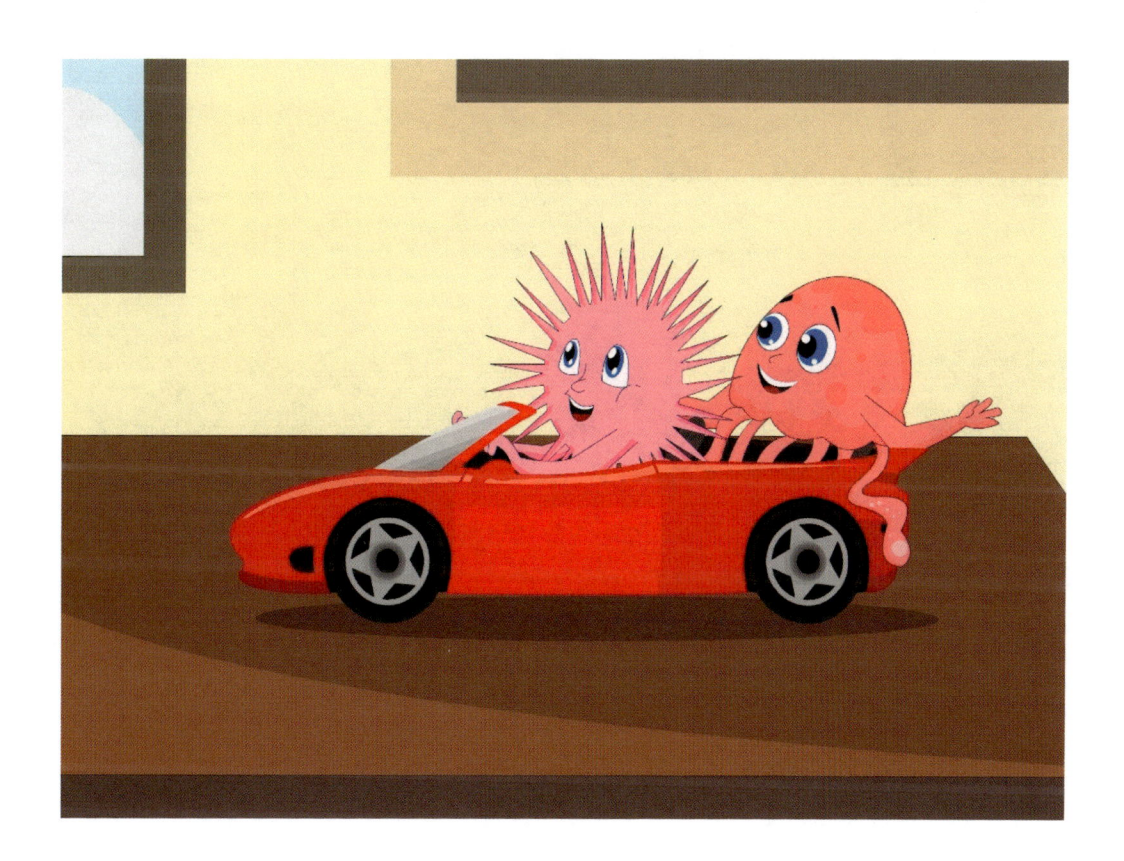

"Finally the last rule!" Jessie Jellyfish chipped in:

"Eat the food you are given, for to waste it is a sin.

Your food is prepared with love and great care,

There may sometimes be things you're not quite sure of in there."

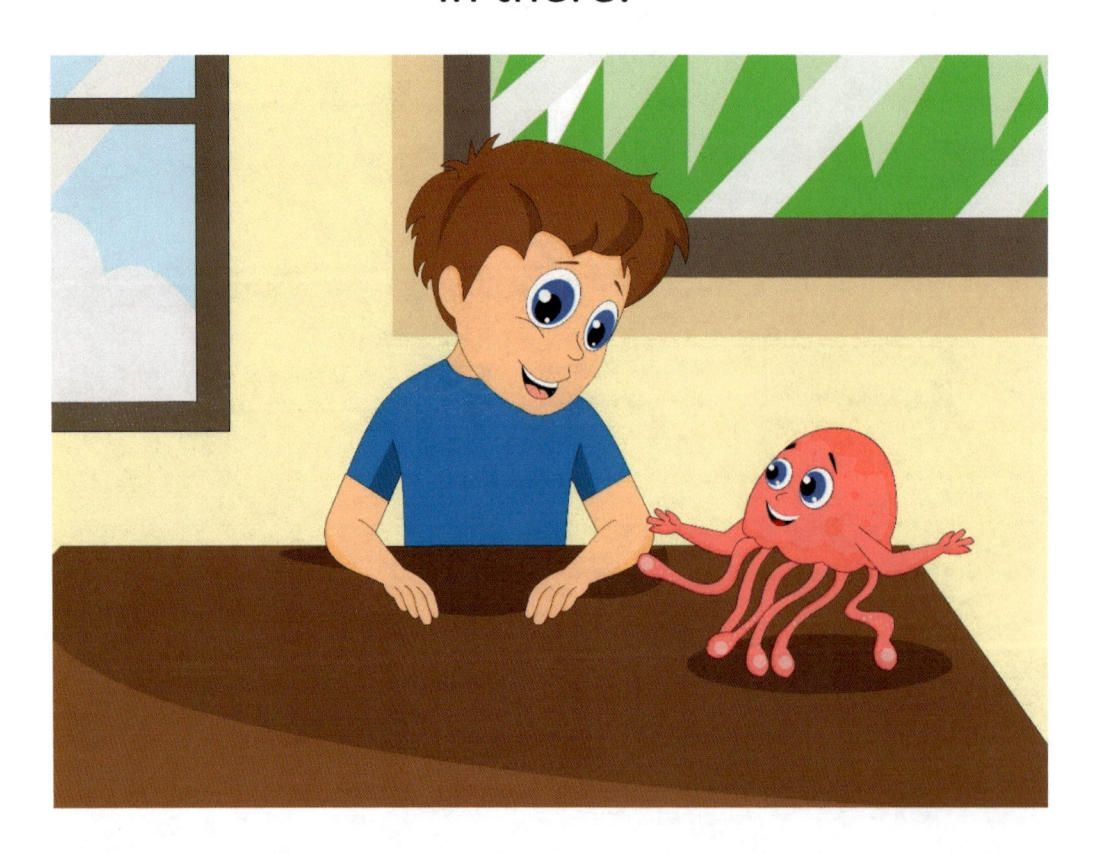

"So try all your food, Oscar, for it is jam-packed full

Of lovely nutrient-rich vitamins and minerals."

"Thank you", said Oscar, "to my wonderful friends,

For showing me the importance eating good food lends."

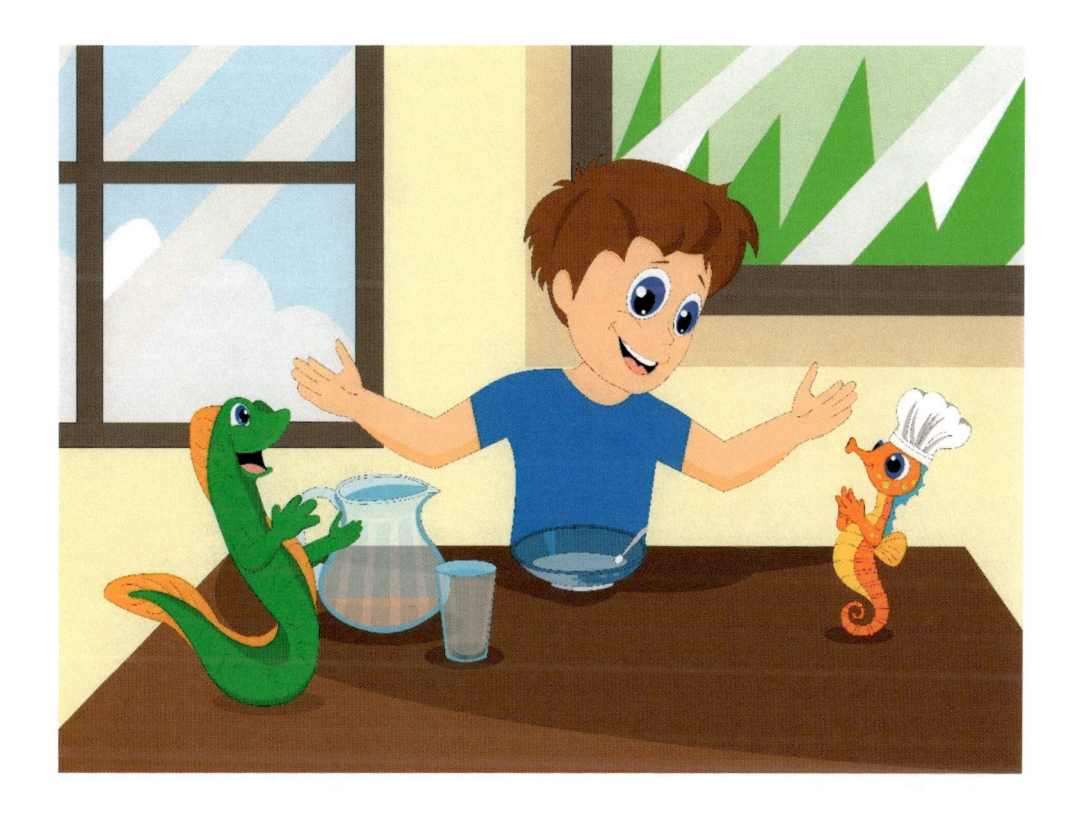

"I understand now that food made for me

Will help me to grow strong, happy and healthy

Choosing my food wisely and with great care and glee

Helps my body to be the optimum me."

About the Author

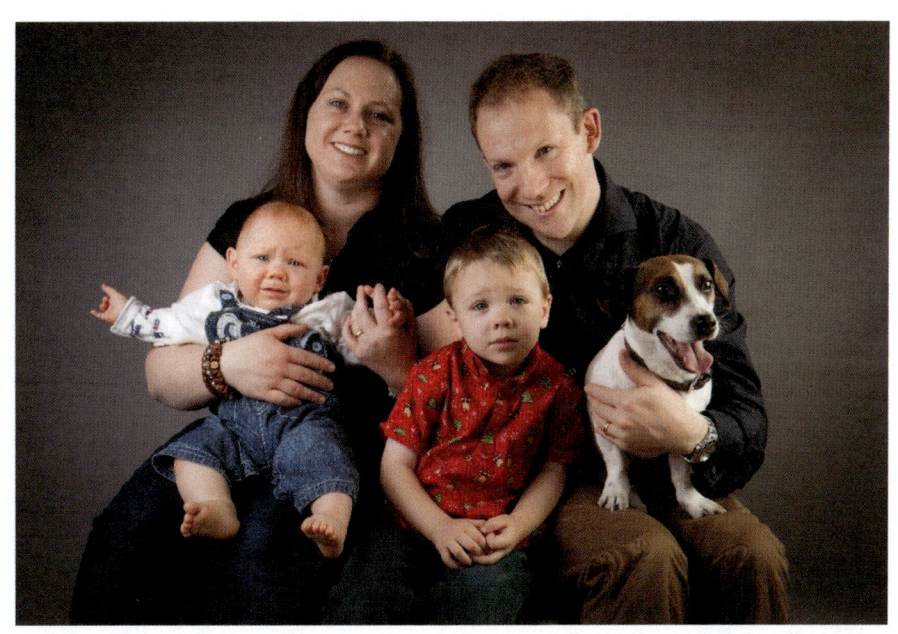

Jo Groenhart first developed Oscar Ocean in 2010. Jo had been working at a thriving wellness centre and noticed that many children didn't realise the importance of stretching or the role this has to play in leading a healthy lifestyle. She noticed on observing infants that they naturally stretch all the time, it's *in their programming*, however as we grow older we lose this good habit. As education is vital in the early years, it makes sense to encourage this good habit and educate our children further.

Oscar Ocean and The Big Stretch was initially produced as a short stretch routine for young children. Shortly after, Jo began to introduce the concept across the 7 habits for health programme, to enable young children to fully engage and begin to take responsibility for their health.

Jo currently lives in Cambridgeshire with her husband Ed, two sons, Isaac and Oakley, and dog, Izzy. Managing their busy family wellness centre and seeing her own client base has given her an ability to help families create their own wellness lifestyle.

Follow the progress of the rest of Oscar's journey at www.facebook.com/jo.groenhart

Josephine NC Groenhart

WEEKLY MEAL PLANNER WEEK 1

	Breakfast	Lunch	Dinner	Snack	Snack
Monday					
Tuesday					
Wednesday					
Thursday					
Friday					
Saturday					
Sunday					

Oscar Ocean and the Big Feast

WEEKLY MEAL PLANNER WEEK 2

	Breakfast	Lunch	Dinner	Snack	Snack
Monday					
Tuesday					
Wednesday					
Thursday					
Friday					
Saturday					
Sunday					

WEEKLY MEAL PLANNER WEEK 3

	Breakfast	Lunch	Dinner	Snack	Snack
Monday					
Tuesday					
Wednesday					
Thursday					
Friday					
Saturday					
Sunday					

WEEKLY MEAL PLANNER WEEK 4

	Breakfast	Lunch	Dinner	Snack	Snack
Monday					
Tuesday					
Wednesday					
Thursday					
Friday					
Saturday					
Sunday					

Josephine NC Groenhart

JOIN OCSAR AND SAMMY IN THEIR NEXT ADVENTURE
OSCAR OCEAN AND THE BIG SLEEP

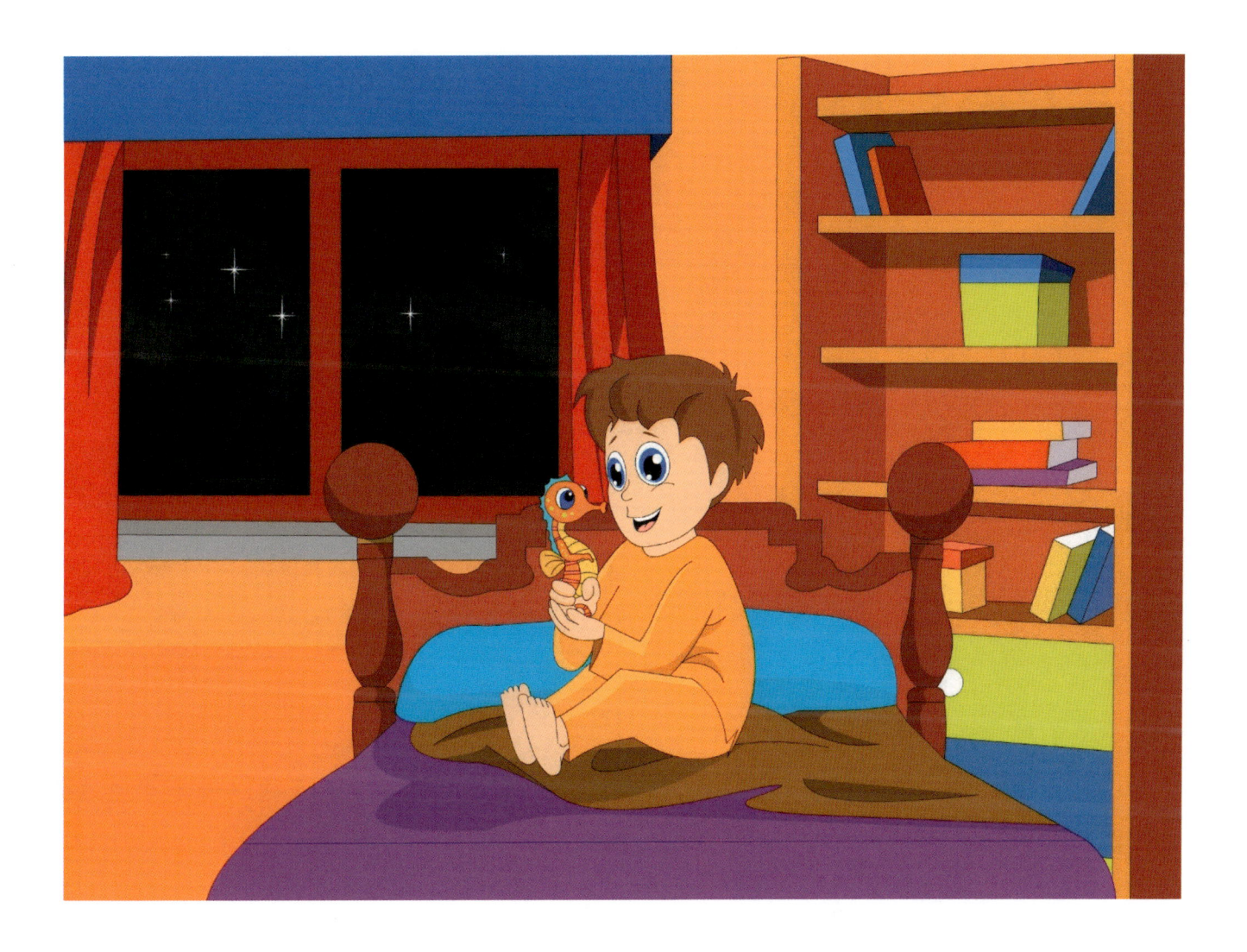

Josephine NC Groenhart

Oscar Ocean and the Big Feast

Josephine NC Groenhart

Made in the USA
Charleston, SC
04 May 2016